Herbal Remedies

Powerful Natural Remedies and Recipes for Health, Wellness, Anti-aging and Beauty

Contents

Chapter 1. The Whys and Hows of Anti-Aging... 1

Chapter 2. Herbs to Help With the Aging Process 9

Chapter 3. Teas That Are Sure to Work 23

Chapter 4. Natural Smoothie Recipes for Anti-Aging 39

Chapter 5. Homemade Anti-Aging Cream Recipes 57

Chapter 6. The Effects of Stress & Herbs to Help... 72

Chapter 7. Anti-Aging Herbal Facemasks 82

Chapter 8. Bonus Anti-Aging Tips................... 98

© **Copyright 2019 by Felix M. White All rights reserved.**

This document is geared toward providing exact and reliable information in regard to the topic and issue covered. The publication is sold with the idea that the publisher is not required to render accounting, officially permitted, or otherwise, qualified services. If advice is necessary, legal or professional, a practiced individual in the profession should be ordered.

- From a Declaration of Principles which was accepted and approved equally by a Committee of the American Bar Association and a Committee of Publishers and Associations.

In no way is it legal to reproduce, duplicate, or transmit any part of this document in either electronic means or in printed format. Recording of this publication is strictly prohibited and any storage of this document is not allowed unless with written permission from the publisher. All rights reserved.

The information provided herein is stated to be truthful and consistent, in that any liability, in terms of inattention or otherwise, by any usage or abuse of any policies, processes, or directions contained within is the solitary and utter responsibility of the recipient reader. Under no circumstances will any legal responsibility or blame be held against the publisher for any reparation, damages, or monetary loss due to the information herein, either directly or indirectly.

Respective authors own all copyrights not held by the publisher.

The information herein is offered for informational purposes solely, and is universal as so. The presentation of the information is without contract or any type of guarantee assurance.

The trademarks that are used are without any consent, and the publication of the trademark is without permission or backing by the trademark owner. All trademarks and brands within this book are for clarifying purposes only and are the owned by the owners themselves, not affiliated with this document.

Chapter 1. The Whys and Hows of Anti-Aging

If you live in the US, it's been proven that most people don't live past the age of eighty. However, that actually isn't many people's main concern. Many people worry about aging gracefully as well as making sure they have a longer life. Anti-aging products are meant to help with one or the other, but natural anti-aging remedies are meant to help with both. There are natural ways to increase the likelihood of living longer as well as aging in a graceful manner.

You may be asking yourself what aging gracefully entails, but it is about the way you look when you age. Some people will look older than they are, and this can show that they've had a harder life or their genetics may be predisposed to aging ungracefully or at a seemingly quicker rate than others.

It's not quite proven why we age, but everyone knows that we cannot be immortal. For life to go on aging will happen, but you can keep your body healthy and keep it from showing the signs of your age a little longer. It's important that you age gracefully in both beauty and strength. You'll want to be healthy when you get older, and the key is to actually start worrying about it when you're young. There are changes that you can make to make sure that you age in a more graceful manner, even if your genetics make you predisposed to do the opposite.

Many people think that our genes will determine how long we live, but there is another theory that over time our DNA is damaged up until the point where we cannot function properly anymore. Either way, you can still make choices to prevent the aging process from taking such a toll on your body.

Anti-aging is about pushing the limits of the aging process to see how you can increase your lifespan and the quality of your life and beauty. Anti-aging creams are usually meant to help with wrinkles, crows-feet, dark spots which are usually caused by age, and sagging of the skin.

Anti-Aging Medication:

There actually is anti-aging medication out there, and it's meant to extend your lifespan and promote your healthspan as well. Your healthspan is how long you can stay healthy despite your age before your health begins to degrade. However, anti-aging medication, prescription wise, is not considered to be something that is common. It is also something that is most likely not to become common. You'll find that like all prescription medications the side effects make it risky. There is another alternative. It has been proven that diet, nutrition and exercise do actually affect the aging process, and it will help to determine how gracefully you age including how long your lifespan is.

Remember the Small Changes:

It's important that you remember the small changes that will affect your aging process as well. For example, alcohol consumption and drug use, including tobacco, can cause the aging process to speed up because it'll take a toll on your skin as well as your organs, mainly your lungs and your liver. As your organs go bad and your health degrades, you'll see the effects of aging much more on your outer beauty. Anti-aging supplements, herbal remedies, and solutions can help to minimize the damage, but it's easier if the damage is not done in the first place.

What most people don't know is that sugar can actually speed up the aging process. It is even known to be a direct cause of aging, and it can significantly decrease your lifespan because of it. Sleep is also known to be extremely important to the aging process because sleep is where your body can rest and recover, and the diet you have and the exercise you do is important because it will affect your internal organs.

Why Worry about Anti-Aging Solutions:

The reason people worry about aging is because people are scared of death and they want to be beautiful. There is a lot of importance put on beauty, especially for women but also for men, by social standards. This is especially true if you live in the US. So skip the over the counter medications, false anti-aging hacks, and any prescription medication.

There's no reason to risk the side effects, and instead you can just worry about increasing your lifespan, keeping your skin and hair looking young, as well as making sure that you live a healthy and quality life. The tips and tricks that you find in this book will help you to keep wrinkles away, your hair shiny, keep away dark spots and live a healthier life overall so that your life is prolonged and the quality goes up.

There's no reason to dread getting older if you have the right solutions that you're using to help you age gracefully. From creams to teas, there are many tools that you can use to make sure that everything goes according to your plan. Start as young as you can, and you'll notice the difference as you get older. Many of these tips and tricks aren't even something that is taxing to add into your daily regime, making it easy to age gracefully and healthily.

Chapter 2. Herbs to Help With the Aging Process

There are many herbal remedies that can help with the aging process, and usually you can get them in just a supplement, but some of them you can actually cook with. It's easy to make sure that you have the right herbs, and some are more common than you think. Remember that fresh herbs can be grown right in your backyard and be used while they're fresh but you can also dry them yourself. Dried herbs should always be properly labeled and stored in a cool, dry place that's out of direct sunlight and in airtight containers to keep moisture from ruining your herbs.

Sage:

Sage is actually found in your spice cabinet most of the time, making it easy to use and even easier to find. It's usually as quick as a trip to the grocery store, and you can usually get it both fresh, in the produce section, and dried in the spice section. It's up to you and the remedy you try. Many people will take a pill made out of sage as well. One of the main reasons that people age is inflammation, but it's not normal inflammation. It's inflammation that reaches a cellular level that causes your body to age even faster than it should.

There are many conditions that you may have that could put you at a risk of this type of inflammation including most types of arthritis, asthma, and the hardening of your arteries. You can add sage into what you're cooking as well, and it's recommended that you to try do that at least once daily for the best results. Most people feel better after adding sage into their regular diet, as it'll keep any and all inflammation down, including from injuries.

Thyme:

You can also find thyme at your local grocery store, but it's also common to find at the flea market or farmer's market if you live in the southern US. Even if you can't get it fresh, you can usually find dried thyme, and it doesn't matter if it's ground fine or not. You should just use it to help with the aging process. Many people suffer from bacterial infections, which can speed the aging process alone, and thyme can help to kill these bacterial infections. It can be something as harmless as a sore throat, but each one will potentially speed the aging process up a little more.

If you can keep yourself healing from infections better, you're much more likely to live healthier and longer. Infections from basic to major will start to take their toll on your body. So speed them along. Many people will even use a thyme tea. Thyme is one of the herbs that is easy to grow in your backyard, so it's rather easy to get fresh. You can usually even grow it in a pot inside.

Italian Spice:

Italian spice is also something that you're most likely going to have in your kitchen cabinet, and you may already cook with it if you're a fan of Italian food. The reason it's anti-aging is because it will help to protect your skin on a cellular level from damage. Just remember that Italian spice is actually a pre-done blend that can help you out. Basil is the key ingredient, and it can help you out on its own as well because basil has a lot of antioxidants that help to repair any damage as well as boost your overall health. Your skin is harmed by free radicals and this blend helps to protect you against it, keeping away dark spots and premature wrinkles.

Turmeric:

Turmeric is a root that can usually be found in your spice cabinet as well, but it's not as commonly used as other spices. It's an herb that is great at helping with inflammation which damages your overall health as well as your skin. It can help with asthma and arthritis as well, and it can even help to protect you from lung cancer by reducing your chances of it, even if you're a smoker.

Many people just take a teaspoon of turmeric a day instead of trying to cook with it, and this is enough to help with the aging process. Other people will mix it with tuna or spice up dishes that are meat based. There are even supplement forms where it can be helpful.

Gymnema Sylvestre:

This isn't an herb that many people are familiar with, but it is one that can help work. The name translates into sugar destroyer, and it is usually taken by chewing a few leaves of the plant. Sugar consumption is one of the main factors that is causing people to die at a young age and their health to degrade, as it's horrible for aging gracefully. It can help to regulate blood sugar levels, which means that it can actually help with diabetes.

Having imbalanced blood sugar can cause man diseases, including heart disease, hyperactivity, insomnia, fatigue, diabetes, and even obesity. If you can cut down your sugar consumption and manage to control your blood sugar levels, which this herb can do, then you'll find it's much easier to age gracefully with this anti-aging herb.

Ginger:

Ginger is a versatile herb, and it's great for anti-aging. It was commonly used in Chinese medicine as well as Ayurvedic medicine. Ginger root can be thick or thin, but it can be used no matter what. You can find it in white, yellow, red, or brown varieties, but all are helpful. You can usually get dried ginger in the spice section of your grocery store. However, if you go to the produce section, ginger root is usually sitting out.

It has many nutrients to it, including copper, vitamin B6, and potassium, manganese, and even magnesium. However, gingerols is where most of its anti-ageing nutrients come from. It helps as an anti-inflammatory, digestive relief, nausea relief, and it even helps to make sure your heart is healthy, which is important if you want to lengthen your lifespan. It will also boost your overall immune system.

Basil:

Basil is a great way to help with anti-aging, and that's because it's full of antioxidants. This is why it helps in the Italian spice blend. Antioxidants are extremely important because they are usually your first line of defense to keep free radicals in check. Free radicals are going to cause and speed along the aging process, and it'll cause dark spots, wrinkles, illness, and even sagging skin. You can cook with basil, drink basil tea, take a basil supplement or use it in so many more ways to make sure that you get all of the antioxidants that will help you with the aging process.

Bilberry:

Bilberry is not something that you'd find commonly in the grocery store, and if you plan to use it you usually have to order it online. However, it is great for anti-aging for the same reason that basil is. Bilberry is packed with tons of antioxidants that are going to help your body stay looking and feeling young throughout the years.

Gingko:

Gingko has also been proven to help the effects of aging by helping your brain get more blood. As you age, your brain is going to start to be affected, and gingko can help with that. It'll help you slow down the effects of aging and keep your mental capacity sharp. It's even been proven to help people that suffer from Alzheimer's disease, and it can even help with other forms of dementia.

Ginseng:

This is commonly known as a Chinese herb, and it's great at making sure that you stay looking young. It helps to tone both your muscles as well as your skin, and it will also improve your appetite, which is great if you're pairing it with the right type of diet to help the aging process as well. It'll help with the digestion of your food which leads to nutrient absorption, and it can even help to restore sexual energy if your libido is suffering.

Peppermint:

Peppermint doesn't just help your digestive system or act as a stimulant. It is also great because of its level of antioxidants that is going to help your system and help fight against the aging process. It'll keep your health up, and it's easy to grow peppermint and even buy it. It can even help to prevent both heart disease and cancer. A lot of age-related disorders can be prevented or helped through the use of peppermint on a regular basis.

Different Ways to Use Them:

There are many ways to use the herbs listed, and they even mix into herbal remedies as well. You don't have to worry about just taking the herb in its pure form. There are many different options for using an herb for its anti-aging benefits, and there are still many herbs that can help. This goes hand in hand with making sure that your diet is proper for keeping you healthy. For example, garlic is great at boosting your immune system, even if it won't' really help the effects of aging on your skin. If you're sick less often, then you're going to look and feel healthier though.

Chapter 3. Teas That Are Sure to Work

There are many teas that can help with the anti-aging process, and you can usually drink them either hot or cold. It's more common to drink the tea hot, and if you are going to drink it cold it'll need to be made in advance and then chilled. Remember to add your sweeten before you chill your tea as it'll mix in better. Try to avoid any and all sugar in your teas, and instead try to use honey. Honey is also important to help keep the effects of aging away, since it is also full of antioxidants and many other nutrients.

Tea #1 Chai & Coconut Blend

If you're a lover of chai tea, then try this coconut blended chai that is full of antioxidants that are sure to help you stay looking young. This tea isn't something that is bland, and it's truly a treat to add to your daily routine, as its rich in both flavor and benefits. It is also great at disease prevention, and the cloves, ginger, cinnamon and even anise is great for helping to make sure you have everything to keep you healthy. The coconut milk is known for its anti-aging benefits as well.

Ingredients:

1. 2 Cups Water, Filtered
2. 1 Tablespoon Chai Tea Mix
3. 2 Whole Star Anise
4. 1 ½ Whole Cardamom Pods, Green
5. 1 ½ Teaspoons Cinnamon
6. 2 Tablespoons Honey, Raw
7. 4-6 Ounces Coconut Milk

Directions:

1. Add the chai mix, spices, and water into a pot and bring it to a simmer. You do not need to bring it to a boil.
2. You can then reduce it to low heat, and then cover it, letting it infuse for at least ten minutes.

3. Then, make sure to strain it all through a mesh to make sure that there are no whole spices still.
4. Add in the coconut milk as desired, and stir in the honey. Stirring in the honey first usually works best because the hotter it is the easier it is to stir.

Tea #2 Pine Needle Tea

Pine needles are actually extremely useful, and they're very favorable for your health. It has a lot of vitamin C, which will help to boost your immune system and keep you healthy when you use it on a regular basis. It also has many antioxidants and even vitamin A. Just remember that you shouldn't just brew any pine needles. It's best to order the right ones, as certain varieties of pine are toxic instead of helpful. The peppermint that is commonly added to this tea, such as in the recipe below, is also added for its antioxidants, just like honey. This is a simple tea that many people love to add in around the holidays when they put other anti-aging teas away.

Ingredients:

1. 2 Teaspoons Pine Needles, Chopped
2. 1 Tablespoon Honey, Raw
3. 1 Teaspoon Peppermint Leaves, Dried

Directions:

1. Bring a full cup of water to a boil, and ten add in your pine needles and peppermint leaves.
2. Reduce the heat to just a simmer, and let the mixture simmer for about five to ten minutes. You should cover it for the best results.

3. Strain out the peppermint leaves and pine needles, and then add honey.
4. Drink while warm or chill to drink later.

Tea #3 Earthy Blend

If you're looking for a more earthy tea, then the basil and sage in this tea is for you. As stated in the previous chapter, both of these herbs can be found in your spice cabinet already, and they're great for aging. Remember to sweeten with honey, but you're also going to want to add a dash of cinnamon because not only is it actually an appetite suppressant, but it can regulate your blood sugar which will help you to slow down the aging process.

Ingredients:

1. ½ Cinnamon Stick
2. 2 Teaspoons Sage, Dried
3. 1 Teaspoon Basil, Dried
4. 1 Tablespoon Honey, Raw

Directions:

1. Just make sure to bring a cup of water to a boil, and then put in all the herbs as you reduce it to a simmer.
2. Cover and let simmer for about eight to ten minutes.
3. Strain out the herbs, and add the honey while it's hot so it mixes better. D

4. It's best to drink it while warm.

Tea #4 Rosehip Tea

Rosehips are actually an herb that can help you as well because they are antibacterial, anti-viral, and anti-inflammatory as well as holding antioxidants. They are great if you are trying to make an anti-aging tea, and it helps to heal both cells as well as tissue, and repairs damage that free radicals produce. They even have vitamins that will help with longevity as well as vitality and generally boost your immune system. It's best to use them with dried orange rind, as it helps to boost the flavor of the tea as well as helping to boost your vitamin C level, which helps with your immune system. This is yet another simple tea, and it doesn't take too long to make.

Ingredients:

1. 2 Teaspoons Orange Peel, Dried
2. 1 ½ Teaspoons Rosehips, Dried
3. 2 Teaspoons Honey

Directions:

1. Boil a single cup of water. Once the water comes to a boil, then you can add in the herbs and reduce it to a simmer. Some people add in the herbs first and

just bring it to a simmer, keeping it there.
2. It should stay at a simmer for five to eight minutes, and then you can strain the herbs out.
3. Once the herbs are strained, then you can add in the honey.
4. Let it cool or drink it hot. It doesn't matter with this anti-aging tea.

Tea #5 Aloe Tea

Aloe is something that you can grow in your own yard, but it's usually best to just buy aloe juice, which is usually in the pharmaceutical aisle of your local grocery store or superstore. Of course, you'll find that you can replace all of the water with aloe juice as well. Make sure that there is no added sugar to the aloe juice, or it won't be healthy. Aloe juice is great for anti-aging. It's meant to make your skin appear younger and it can help to reduce your wrinkles as well. Add in peppermint and sage for a great drink. Remember to top with honey.

Ingredients:

1. 6 Ounces Aloe Juice
2. 4 Ounces Water
3. 1 Teaspoon Peppermint, Dried
4. ½ Teaspoon Sage, Dried
5. 1 Teaspoon Honey, Raw

Directions:

1. Start by boiling the water, and then reduce it to a simmer after adding sage and peppermint.
2. Let simmer for about eight to ten minutes, and then strain.
3. Add in the honey, and top with aloe juice and drink.

Tea #6 Rosemary Tea

This is an herb that you can find dried easily in your grocery store or grow right in your backyard. Rosemary has many health benefits, and it's commonly used with sage to get an earthy tea that tastes great with honey. It's anti-inflammatory and anti-bacterial, as well as it has immune boosting qualities as well. It is known to stimulate the regeneration of your cells, making you look younger and reducing the effects of aging on your skin. It will help reduce swelling and sagging in your skin as well. Rosemary even helps with your overall skin tone.

Ingredients:

1. 2 Tablespoons Rosemary
2. 1 Tablespoon Sage
3. 2 Teaspoons Honey

Directions:

1. Put all the herbs into a cup of water in a large saucepan, and bring it to a simmer.
2. Keep it simmering for ten to twelve minutes while covered.
3. Strain out all of the herbs, and add in the honey while warm.
4. This tea is best to drink when warm, but you can still drink it cooled if preferred.

Drink Regularly:

The best way to make sure that these teas work is to drink them on a regular basis. You won't always be able to drink them daily, but you can switch it up. Even just taking a simple basil, rosehip, or even orange rind tea will help with the effects of aging. Strive to drink at least once of these teas every day, and it will help to make sure that the effects of aging aren't taking their toll on both your inner and outer body. If you're not drinking anti-aging teas on a regular basis, then you aren't going to reap the benefits of them. They do have immediate benefits, but anti-aging benefits require time.

Chapter 4. Natural Smoothie Recipes for Anti-Aging

There are many smoothie recipes that you can add in to your daily regime for their anti-aging benefits as well. It's great if you're not a tea person, and it keeps you from having to go to herbal supplements. Just remember that many of these smoothies can be tweaked to your tastes, but remember why the ingredients are important in the first place.

Smoothie #1 Tropical Blend

This tropical blend is great if you're worried about the look of your skin and the effect that aging has on it. You don't need to worry anymore, and you already know that both ginger and turmeric powder are great to help repair the damage that the aging process does to your body, and instead it can slow down the aging process. They both also have anti-inflammatory benefits. The pineapple is added because it is high in vitamin C, helping to boost your immune system and slow down aging as well.

It even has bromelain which is known to help detoxify your body, which is also better for aging. The coconut water is also great for anti-aging, as the zinc, iodine, boron, and manganese will act as antioxidants helping to keep your skin looking bright. The banana helps because of the potassium, which will help your muscles keep from losing their tone from the aging process as well. The vanilla is mostly added for flavor.

Ingredients:

1. 1 ½ Teaspoons Ginger, Chopped & Peeled
2. ¾ Cup Coconut Water, Frozen
3. 1 Cup Pineapple, Chopped
4. 1 Cup Banana, Frozen & Sliced
5. 1 Teaspoon Vanilla Extract
6. ¼ Teaspoon Turmeric Powder
7. 2 Teaspoons Honey

Directions:

1. Blend the ginger and vanilla extract first.
2. Then add in all the other ingredients, blending until it's smooth.

Smoothie #2 Blueberry Blend

If you like blueberries, then you're in for a treat. Blueberries are high in antioxidants, which you already know will help you with aging. It's going to help your skin look all the smoother, helping to avoid wrinkles. The almond milk is also good for aging as well as your skin. It's going to help you to look younger even as you grow old, making your aging process graceful. This is a simple smoothie recipe that only needs sweetened with honey. Make sure to freeze your almond milk in advance so that you can have a thick smoothie.

Ingredients:

1. 2 Cups Blueberries, Frozen
2. 2 Tablespoons Honey, Raw
3. 1 Cup Almond Milk, Frozen

Directions:

1. Just blend all ingredients together, and then you can drink.

Smoothie #3 Blackberry Twist

If you like blackberries, this is the smoothie for you, and it has hidden ingredients that are sure to help you boost your immune system as well as help with the aging process. Blackberries are known for their antioxidants, much like blueberries. They are both in the bramble family, but acai powder is also used in this smoothie recipe.

Acai powder is high in both fiber and antioxidants. The fiber helps your system by keeping you healthy and regular, and the honey helps as well. With a few sprigs of rosemary, this is a healthy anti-aging smoothie recipe that won't disappoint. Milk can help to combat heart disease and stroke, and provides needed vitamins to your body.

Ingredients:

1. ½ Cup Whole Milk
2. ¼ Cup Ice
3. 1 Cup Blackberries, Frozen
4. 2 Teaspoons Rosemary, Dried
5. 2 Teaspoons Honey, Raw
6. 1 Teaspoon Acai Powder

Directions:

1. Add in ingredients, and blend until smooth. If you want it thicker, add more milk or ice. If you want it sweeter, then add more honey.

Smoothie #4 Peachy Perfect

Peaches aren't good for anti-aging exactly, but you'll find that they are full of vitamins that your body needs. Peaches do have some antioxidants, but they are not as high as some fruit such as blueberries. The chia seeds will also help to make sure that you have the antioxidants that you need as well as fiber and calcium. The almond milk makes it creamy, and it's good for aging as well, as previously discussed. The spinach keeps you healthy and your brain sharp, which you can lose in the aging process.

Ingredients:

1. 1 ½ Cups Frozen Peaches
2. 2 Tablespoons Honey
3. 1 Tablespoon Chia Seeds
4. ½ Cup Almond Milk, Frozen
5. ¼ Cup Baby Spinach

Directions:

1. Take the honey, baby spinach, and chia seeds first. Blend until smooth.
2. Add in all other ingredients, and continue to blend until smooth.

Smoothie #5 Chocolate Surprise

Chocolate is actually age defying, so long as it's dark chocolate. That's why this smoothie has cocoa powder that will help you to look and feel younger as you get older. Add in a little blueberries for their antioxidants, and then add in a half a cup of almond milk and a little more acai powder to make sure that you have everything you need. Top it all off with sweet honey to make the concoction delightful.

Ingredients:

1. 3 Tablespoons Cocoa Powder
2. 2 Teaspoons Honey, Raw
3. 1 ½ Teaspoons Acai Powder
4. 1 Cup Blueberries, Frozen
5. 1 Cup Vanilla Almond Milk

Directions:

1. Mix everything together and blend until smooth. Add more cocoa powder and honey if you want a sweeter and more prominent taste of chocolate in your smoothie recipe.

Smoothie #6 Strawberry Watermelon Splash

Both strawberries and watermelons are great when you're trying to create an anti-aging smoothie. It's due to the antioxidants, but they have many other benefits as well. Remember that a lot of the berries are safe to use if you're looking for something that will help to make you feel a little healthier. It's also refreshing during a hot day, and it's commonly used in summer. The added peppermint helps a little more for anti-aging while still making sure that it keeps that cool and crisp refreshing taste. Strawberries are high in vitamin C as well as antioxidants. It'll keep your skin looking firm as well as banish any wrinkles that may be trying to form. Watermelon is great to help you keep away from skin discoloration and even to prevent wrinkles.

Ingredients:

1. 2 Cups Seedless Watermelon, Fresh & Cubed
2. 1 Teaspoon Peppermint Extract
3. 1 Cup Frozen Strawberries, Chopped
4. 2 Teaspoons Honey, Raw
5. ¼ Cup Ice

Directions:

1. Add in all ingredients together, and then you can mix until it's smooth. Add more ice if necessary to make it thicker. With frozen fruit, it shouldn't be necessary.

Smoothie #7 Purple Power

The main ingredient to this smoothie is grapes, and that's because grapes are great for anti-aging. They have manganese and vitamin C, and when these are together, it helps to prevent the damage on your skin from ultraviolet radiation, and its antioxidants helps your skin. Add in bananas because of its vitamin B6 and C, which helps with the aging process as well. The almond milk, as discussed, helps as well, but frozen cherry juice also helps. However, it has to be tart cherry juice which is commonly referred to as the ultimate antioxidant solution. You'll need a little more honey in this recipe than usual, though.

Ingredients:

1. 3 Tablespoons Honey
2. ½ Cup Cherry Juice, Frozen
3. ½ Banana, Frozen & Sliced
4. 1 Cup Almond Milk, Cooled
5. 1 Cup Grapes, Frozen

Directions:

1. Mix everything together in the blender, making sure to blend until it's smooth. Make sure the honey is mixed throughout.

Make it Regular:

Smoothies are great for your health, especially when you're adding only whole ingredients. Do not replace it with fruit juice or two percent milk. You need to stick to whole fruits, and you can even freeze fresh fruits so that they have more nutrients than flash frozen fruits. Try not just to add it into your daily routine. Instead, you're going to want to replace one of your meals with these smoothies. Many people will do so for lunch or breakfast. This will also help you to regulate your weight and give you the vitamins you need to stay healthy.

Chapter 5. Homemade Anti-Aging Cream Recipes

There are many different anti-aging creams out there, but they're usually expensive and not worth the money that you're paying. Anti-aging creams are easy to make for yourself, and most of the ingredients are actually easy to get ahold of. So make your own anti-aging creams and know exactly what is being put onto your skin.

Cream #1 Soothing Anti-Aging Cream

This is a cream that primarily uses rose and aloe, and it's a great way to make sure that you have everything you need to banish wrinkles. The rosehip oil works for the same reason that rosehips work for, and the shea butter an jojoba oil will help to make sure that your skin is moisturized and looking younger. The aloe will help to make sure that your skin is healed at a cellular level, and the stearic acid is an emulsifier.

Ingredients:

1. 10-15 Drops Rose Essential Oil
2. 4-6 Drops Lavender Essential Oil
3. ¼ Cup Aloe Juice
4. 1 Tablespoons Beeswax, Grated
5. 1 ½ Tablespoons Shea Butter

6. 1 Tablespoon Rosehip Seed Oil
7. 2 Tablespoons Jojoba Oil

Directions:

1. Start by combining the jojoba oil and the shea butter with the stearic acid and the beeswax. It will need heat, and it's best to put it over a double boiler to melt it. Don't add the rosehip seed oil yet.
2. Make sure everything is melted together, and don't leave it in the heat too long. If you overheat your shea butter, then it will become grainy.
3. The mixture should be poured into a bowl, and then you can stir in the

rosehip seed oil. Wait for it to cool to room temperature.
4. Drizzle in the aloe and then mix it in as well as the essential oils.
5. Pour into glass jars with an airtight seal, and put it in the refrigerator. It has no preservatives, so it should only last three weeks. So make small batches.

Cream #2 Night Cream

This anti-aging cream is better as a night cream, and you just rub it in small circular motions into your skin before you go to bed. You don't have to wash it off, and it's great for anti-aging. The bentonite clay will help to remove impurities and toxin by absorbing them form your skin. The vitamin E oil will block the free radicals which will help you to slow down the aging process, and it can even help with scar tissue. The aloe vera gel will brighten your skin and make you look younger while neutralizing free radicals and repairing any damage to your skin.

It can even help with wrinkles. The almond oil is great to decrease any puffiness around your eyes and dark circles. Lemon essential oil is known as a brightener, which will make you appear younger, and it'll help to detoxify your skin. Raw shea butter is a great moisturizer as well.

Ingredients:

1. 2 Tablespoons Almond Oil
2. 1 Teaspoon Coconut Oil
3. ½ Teaspoon Beeswax, Grated
4. ½ Teaspoon Shea Butter, Organic
5. 1 ½ Teaspoons Vitamin E Oil
6. 1 ½ Teaspoons Honey, Raw
7. ½ Teaspoon Bentonite Clay
8. 8-10 Drops Lemon Essential Oil

Directions:

1. Make sure to use a double boiler to melt the beeswax, coconut oil, almond oil, as well as the shea butter together. Make sure not to overheat it so the shea butter does not become grainy. You will want it to be creamy so it goes on smooth.
2. Take another bowl, and mix in the aloe vera gel, the vitamin E oil, honey, as well as the lemon essential oil.
3. When the beeswax oil is completely cooled it should have the texture of lip balm. You can then break it up and add it to the aloe mixture.
4. Place it into a blender, and continue to blend until it's fully combined.
5. Put it in another bowl, and make sure it's non-metal. Add in the bentonite clay and

stir. It should never come in contract with metal.
6. Place it into a glass jar, and store in a cool and dry place.

Cream #3 Simple Cream

Rosewater is a great toner that is going to make your skin look better, and you're going to find that honey moisturizes your skin. Its antioxidants also work to help reverse and slow down the aging process as well. The almond oil is known to help reverse the aging process as well, and the beeswax is what helps to give it the texture that you need. Grated beeswax is known to melt easier, making the process a little quicker.

Ingredients:

1. 4 Ounces Rose Water
2. 200 Millimeters Almond Oil
3. 1 Teaspoon Raw Honey
4. 8 Teaspoons Beeswax

Directions:

1. Take the beeswax, honey, and almond oil together in a double boiler and melt it on low heat. Make sure the mixture is completely melted and blended all the way through.

2. Then, add in the rosewater one drop at a time. It should turn it into a lotion like texture. Store in an airtight container, but don't close it until it's cooled down.

Cream #4 Wrinkle Cream

Wrinkles are one of the main issues for people who are worried about aging, and this anti-wrinkle cream will help you to keep from forming wrinkles as well as to get rid of any that you may currently have. Essential oils are great for beauty products, and myrrh as well as frankincense have been used since Egyptian times for beauty care regimens because they are great to make your skin look healthy as well as glowing.

Ingredients:

1. ½ Cup Shea butter
2. 5-8 Drops Myrrh Essential Oil
3. 4-6 Drops Lemon Essential Oil
4. 20 Drops Frankincense Essential Oil
5. 2 Tablespoons Coconut Oil

Directions:

1. The coconut oil and shea butter should be put into a bowl, and then you're going to want to whip it until it's light and fluffy, as well as smooth.

2. Then, combine all the essential oils into the mixture.
3. Make sure you have an airtight container ready to store it in. it should be applied after washing your face and patting it dry on a daily basis.

Cream #5 A Simple Eye Cream

If you're using an eye cream, you're probably spending too much money. This is an eye cream that will do anything that an expensive one can, as well as it's easy to make. You don't have to worry about the cost anymore, and it'll keep your eyes from getting puffy or dark. Primrose is a great way to take care of fine lines as well as dark circles. It even makes your skin softer, keeps away irritation, and reduces any inflammation. The coconut oil will moisturize your skin and hydrates it.

Ingredients:

1. ½ Cup Coconut Oil
2. 1 Teaspoon Vitamin E Oil
3. 1 Tablespoon Primrose Oil

Directions:

1. Take the coconut oil, and put it into a microwave safe bowl. Heat it for just fifteen seconds.

2. Mix in the vitamin E oil, making sure it's mixed together.
3. Add in the primrose oil, making sure it's thoroughly mixed.
4. Then put it in an airtight container, storing it in the fridge until it's solid.
5. Once it's solid, you can store it in your medicine cabinet.

Remember the Routine:

Anti-aging creams are a great way to make sure that the immediate signs of aging will help to disappear. Of course, you have to use it on a regular basis for it to really work. You will notice a small difference from one use. However, most people don't notice a difference until they've used it for about a week continuously. As time goes on, more of a difference will be seen, and your skin should take on a healthy tone and glow from using it on a regular basis. You do not need to wash off these creams, and you should let them soak in. remember to apply liberally.

Chapter 6. The Effects of Stress & Herbs to Help

Everyone has heard that worrying too much can cause wrinkles, and it's true. Stress speeds along the aging process, and if you want to live a long, healthy life where your beauty stays intact, you're going to want to make sure that you're living a life where your stress is managed. You don't have to manage your stress with over the counter medications or prescription drugs, and instead you can manage them in a natural way with different herbs. These herbs can be used as supplements or in tincture or tea form.

Taking this as a supplement or tea is most common. Make sure that your doctor is aware if you plan to take an herb to help you manage your stress because they will tell you if it is safe with any medical conditions you may have or with any medications you may be taking. You will also need to list any over the counter medications that you may have. Of course, most herbs are safe to take for stress, and it's rare that they could cause dangers as they are known for having less side effects than prescription or over the counter drugs.

The Effects of Stress:

Stress will affect your sleep, and it can even give you heart and digestive issues, such as stomach ulcers and strokes. Of course, you need to minimize your stress if you want to avoid these issues. It is important that stress does not actually reduce your sleep as it can lead to many different diseases and illnesses. It will start to affect your everyday life as well.

Stress can also wreck your appearance, and one of the ways is because your body will produce more oil, which can lead to blackhead and acne. This can make you look older than you are, but it can also cause your hair to thin. Stress can cause fine lines and wrinkles, which you can help to combat with these herbs as well as the creams seen in the previous chapter.

Chamomile:

Chamomile is one of the biggest ways that you can reduce stress, and the most common way to use it is in a chamomile tea. Remember that it can make you sleepy, so it's best that you do it before bed. You can even use it in a chamomile bath to make sure that you are getting the full benefits of what chamomile has to offer for your skin and hair. It's a mild sedative, and it'll help to increase your quality and quantity of sleep which will help you to manage stress naturally as well. Sleep is a great time for your body to sort out the stress of the day, and you even get to do this mentally via dreaming. It's even known to help people who are suffering from anxiety disorders.

Passionflower:

Passionflower is also a sedative, but it's great at calming your nerves. When you use it in a supplement or a tea, then you're more likely to just get a little sleepy than too sleepy. It has extreme calming properties, which will put you in a tranquil state. It can even help to stave off anxiety and even depression. However, you should always keep in mind that passionflower does not create grogginess, unlike prescription medications that work in a similar manner. It's great at calming an anxiety attack as well.

Lemon Balm:

Lemon balm is yet another herb that can help you to make sure that you're managing your stress in a natural way without medication. It's even easy to grow in your own backyard. It has been used since the time of the Middle Ages to help with stress and even anxiety, including anxiety and stress disorders. When used on a regular basis, it can even stave off anxiety attacks. You can take it as a capsule, tincture, or a tea, but a tea or capsule is usually the most common way to take it. You should be able to find a capsule at your local health store.

Lavender:

Lavender is easy to grow in your backyard, and it can help with any anxiety or stress as well, so you can say goodbye to wrinkles caused by stress. Just growing it in your backyard can be helpful because of the aromatherapy qualities, so if you are growing it, just keep your windows open before harvesting it. You can dry it and use it in your food as well as a tea. You can get it in capsules, but you can also make your own tincture. You can even just get a lavender essential oil and rub it on your temples to decrease stress, and it'll even help you to get rid of headaches and migraines as well. It's known to stabilize your moods and center yourself just from the smell.

Peppermint:

The smell of peppermint is known to help you with your stress as well, and you've already learned that peppermint is a great source of antioxidants. That's why it's recommended that you use it as a tea that you sip at slowly when you're trying to use it for its anxiety relieving properties as well. However, you can always just get peppermint essential oil and rub it on your temples like you would lavender oil, and that will help as well. It can even have the added benefit of calming your upset stomach or nausea, no matter if it's digested or not.

Rosemary:

Rosemary tea has already been explored in this book as a great anti-aging agent when taken as a tea, but it will also help to keep your stress in check. You don't always have to use it as a tea, as you can use it as an essential oil as well. It's also great for essential oil, and you can just have it in a bath if you're desiring to decrease your stress either.

Use it Regularly:

It doesn't matter how you're using these herbs. Just remember that using them on a regular basis is usually the best way to make sure it's effective. You can choose the aromatherapy route, the tea route, or use a capsule. Many of these can even be put into a bath to help you relieve your stress, and hot baths are known to help you with your stress as well, especially if relaxing candles are lit around you. A hot bath will relax your muscles.

Another way to help reduce your stress in a natural manner is to make sure that you're exercising regularly as it helps you to physically work out your stress, and yoga or Tai Chi will help because it's a mixture of centering yourself and exercising. However, simple meditation with aromatherapy oils, such as some listed above, can help as well.

Chapter 7. Anti-Aging Herbal Facemasks

Facemasks are a great way to help you if you're dealing with the visual effects of aging. Just make sure to get rid of those dark spots, fine lines, and wrinkles. You don't need to deal with crows-feet any longer, and there's no reason that you actually need to look your age. There are many different ingredients that you can use, and you don't need expensive ingredients all the time. It's usually best if you're switching up facemasks so that you can get all the benefits each one has to offer, but each and every facemask will help to make sure that your skin is wrinkle free, soft, and glowing just like when you were younger.

Facemask #1 Egg Wash for Eyes

You'll see the effects of aging at your eyes first on your face, so trying to find a way to reduce that is usually best. It's important that your eye mask has a natural astringent, which are what the egg whites are for. It'll make your skin look firmer and even tighter, which gives you the younger look you're going for. The aloe is going to help with dark circles and puffiness as well.

Ingredients:

1. 2 Egg Whites
2. 1 Teaspoon Aloe Vera

Directions:

1. Just beat the egg whites and the aloe together.
2. Gently brush on the egg wash, and let it sit for five to eight minutes.
3. The mixture should completely dry before you wash it off with cool water. Pat the area dry, and do not dry it roughly or it will cause harm to the area.

Facemask #2 Dark Spot Eliminator

If you're looking for a way to get rid of dark spots, then this is the facemask for you. Once again, it's a facemask that is inexpensive and easy to make. It's even easier to use. The calamine lotion is going to sooth your skin and absorb any oil that is on it, and the tea tree oil is anti-inflammatory as well as anti-bacterial. This will take care of any acne as well as puffiness, and the lemon juice will help to lighten your skin and adjust pH.

Ingredients:

1. 4 Ounces Calamine Lotion
2. 35-40 Drops Tea Tree Oil
3. 1 Tablespoons Lemon Juice, Fresh

Directions:

1. Take a clean bowl, pouring in the calamine lotion and then add in the tea tree oil. Make sure it's mixed together.
2. Then, you can add the lemon juice, but make sure that there are no seeds there.
3. Pour the liquid mixture into a bottle, and make sure to shake it well.

4. You can refrigerate it for use, but when you do use it, just apply it to the skin and wait for it to dry on your skin. Leave it for another five minutes.
5. Wash with cool water, and then pat the area dry.

Facemask #3 Wrinkle Free Facemask

Say goodbye to all of your wrinkles and fine lines. You don't need to worry about any sagging skin with this wonderful and easy facemask. It doesn't even require that many ingredients, so it's cheap and easy to make. Retinol is a wrinkle fighting ingredient that can be found in carrots, which is why they're in this facemask. You'll find that your skin is instantly tightened with the egg whites. The aloe will help to moisturize your skin, and that will give it that soft glow you're looking for.

Ingredients:

1. 1 Teaspoon Aloe Vera
2. 1 Egg White
3. 1 ½ Tablespoons Carrot, Shredded

Directions:

1. Make sure to shred your carrots fine, and you can use a peeler to do it as well. It'll help you to get thin shredded pieces.

2. Beat your aloe and egg white together, and then add in your carrots.
3. Make sure to mix well, and apply it to your face.
4. Make sure to apply it to your face generously, and let it dry.
5. It should sit for eight to ten minutes, and then you can wash it off with cool water. Never dry your face harshly. It's usually best to just pat it dry.

Facemask #4 Facial Lifter & Cleanser

Summer is a great time until you realize just how much the sun speeds up the aging process, and there's no reason to deal with it. You help to heal your delicate skin and look younger, smoother, and fresher. The yogurt in this recipe has lactic acid, and that will soften and sooth your skin. It'll even help you with collagen production, and the honey is going to moisturize your skin while containing antioxidants and antibacterial properties. The vitamin E is going to help to heal any damage that has been done already, and the lemon will remove the oil and brighten your overall look, helping to remove dark spots from your skin.

Ingredients:

1. 1 Cup Greek Yogurt
2. 3 Tablespoons Honey, Raw
3. ½ Teaspoon Vitamin E Oil
4. 1 ½ Teaspoons Lemon Juice, Fresh

Directions:

1. Just mix everything together. If you are making it in a large batch, remember to keep it in the fridge. There are no preservatives in this facemask, making it better for your skin. Only keep it for up to five days.
2. Apply it liberally to your face, and then let it sit for fifteen to twenty minutes.
3. Wash off with cool water, and then pat dry.

Facemask #5 Traditional Turmeric

Turmeric has already been discussed to be helpful for anti-aging, and a Turmeric facemask has been used for centuries in Chinese and Indian traditions. It'll help to reduce any redness or inflammation which will actually cause wrinkles and puffiness that is going to cause fine lines. The turmeric mask will take care of that before it even starts and help to repair lines or wrinkles that are already there. Its antioxidants are going to help to rejuvenate your skin as well. Milk and honey is known to soften and rejuvenate your skin as well, making sure the turmeric does not irritate it.

Ingredients:

1. 1 ½ Teaspoon Honey, Raw
2. 1 Teaspoon Whole Milk

3. 1 ½ Teaspoons Turmeric

Directions:

1. Make sure to mix everything together in a clean bowl.
2. Apply it to your skin, and let it dry. The honey and turmeric will have it dry despite the milk.
3. Leave it for ten to twelve minutes before washing and patting dry. Remember to use cool water.

Facemask #6 Blended Chocolate Mask

This is an anti-aging facemask that you can make right in your blender, and it's going to help to make sure that you stay looking young and refreshed. The avocado is going to help because of the Omega-3s in it, and it's going to moisturize your skin and help control free radical damage. It has vitamin E and antioxidants in it already. The cocoa is going to provide even more antioxidants, and it'll even balance your hormones to help you age gracefully. The almond milk is going to hydrate your skin as well as give you more vitamin E to help with any sun damage, and the green tea is going to iron out any wrinkles or lines you have. It'll help inflammation, and that's because it's full of polyphenols.

Ingredients:

1. ½ Cup Almond Milk, Unsweetened
2. 1 Teaspoon Matcha Green Tea
3. 3 ½ Tablespoons Raw Cocoa Powder
4. 1 Small Avocado, Ripe & Peeled

Directions:

1. Make sure that your avocado is peeled, ripe, cut up, and the seed is out of the way.
2. Put all of your ingredients into a blender, and make sure to mix it until it's completely smooth.

3. Apply it liberally to your face, and let it sit for fifteen to twenty minutes. It's safe and tasty to eat any leftovers in the meantime as well. So it's good for your face and your stomach.
4. Then, you'll want to wash it with cool water, and it should be patted dry.

Facemask Tips:

It's best not to make your facemask up in advance unless it's just a day or two. This is because you'll have to worry about it going bad if the fridge stays open too long or the container isn't right. There is no preservatives or chemicals in these facemasks, but that's the exact reason you'll find that they work so well to keep the effects of aging from being seen, helping you to age gracefully and beautifully. You can use any of these facemasks once a day, and using it daily is going to help you look even better and younger. You can even apply it to your neck to make sure the skin doesn't get too lose. It's best to do this with the facemasks that have egg whites because as you get older it's an easier for the skin to get looser here.

Chapter 8. Bonus Anti-Aging Tips

There are some more anti-aging natural tips that will help you to make sure that you have control on how old you look. You don't have to let your genetics decide everything for you, and you don't need to turn to chemical laden products to keep you looking and feeling younger. The natural remedies that you've found so far are going to help to make sure that you don't' just look younger but you are actually as healthy as you were in your younger years as well if not healthier. These tips are going to help you reach the same goal.

Anti-Aging Supplements:

There are some anti-aging supplements that you can take as well. They aren't just for anti-aging. Instead, they're just great to help make sure that you stay healthy, and their anti-aging benefits are nothing to laugh at.

Fish Oil: The Omega-3 in fish oil is great, and it's a cheap supplement that you can get at any health store and usually even a grocery store. It will help you to prevent your skin from looking aged and wrinkled. It can even prevent fine lines.

Polypodium Leucotomos Extract: This is great to protect you against sagging skin, which often comes with age as well as discoloration. It can even help with sun damage which will speed the ageing process along. It's great to restore collagen, and it'll combat any problems with wrinkles. You'll need to take 500mg, and it's best that you take it before sun exposure for the day.

Vitamin C: Vitamin C is actually a great anti-aging supplement as well. It will protect your skin from looking dull, and it can even protect against fine lines and wrinkles. It's best to take vitamin C every day. However, you don't just have to take a pill. You can use topical vitamin C, but many people find the capsule to be a little easier. It'll help your cells to regenerate, making the damage that aging does a little less.

Vitamin E: Remember that vitamin E doesn't just have to be applied topically. You already know that it can help with wrinkles, sagging, and even discoloration, but it doesn't have to be taken internally. You can apply the oil externally, and this will help you to target the areas that you're worried about the most.

Coenzyme Q10: This is best for wrinkles, and it's very similar to vitamin C as well as vitamin E. It'll help with your overall health, but a little more importantly for this it'll help with your skin. It'll help reduce the cellular damage that you're experiencing, and its antioxidant rich. It's considered to be a youth-booster, and it can start helping you in as little as two weeks.

Glucosamine: This is a supplement that is sure to help you with your skin that's sagging and any fine lines that you may be experiencing. It's a topical ingredient, and it has amino acid. However, it does help when taken internally as well. It will start reducing your wrinkles and fine lines within two weeks, and it'll accelerate your healing as well. Your skin will even be a little more hydrated, helping it to look younger and have a glow about it.

A Few More Tips:

There is still more that you can do naturally to make sure that you're not experiencing the side effects of aging as roughly. Anti-aging doesn't have to just be an application. It can be a lifestyle, and it'll help you to increase your lifespan and your healthspan as well. Lifestyle changes, such as taking a tea or a smoothie a day with facemasks and helpful herbs in your food is going to help you. Remember that sleep and exercise is going to help as well, and there are many helpful foods and spices that have already been stated that will help you with anti-aging. Of course, you can also add a little more olive oil into your diet as well.

Extra virgin olive oil is usually best, and that's because it's a healthy fat that is going to make your skin shine. Nuts are also going to help, and they have anti-aging fats, minerals and even vitamins. Cashews, peanuts, almonds and walnuts are predominantly the best, and they can be added as a healthy snack. It'll even help to keep you away from junk food which has the sugar that would cause issues and speed the aging process along.

Making a lifestyle with it all is the best way to age gracefully, and start as early as you can. Some people get wrinkles when they're sixty but some get them when they're thirty. You can see the effects of aging at any age, and your lifestyle will make a difference. These natural solutions can make the difference in how the aging process affects you.